A GUIDE TO JUICING HEALTH

GOD'S DESIGN FOR THE HUMAN BODY
A DEVOTIONAL AND RECIPE BOOK

BY DAPHNE GRESHAM-GADDY

TABLE OF CONTENTS

TABLE OF CONTENTS CONT.

- How cold press juicing can improve digestion, immunity, and energy levels
- Incorporating cold press juices into a balanced diet

Chapter 5: Recipes for Cold Press Juices
- Refreshing citrus blends
- Green detox juices
- Nutrient-packed fruit and vegetable combinations
- Immunity-boosting elixirs

Chapter 6: Incorporating Juicing into a Long-Term Healthy Lifestyle
- Creating a juicing routine that fits your schedule
- Tips for meal planning and incorporating cold press juices into meals and snacks
- Sustaining a healthy lifestyle with cold press juicing

Chapter 7: Types of Juicers

Chapter 8: The Advantage of the Cold Press Juicer

INTRODUCTION:

Welcome to Cold Press Juicing: A Comprehensive Guide to Juicing Health. In this book, you will discover the benefits of cold press juicing, learn about different techniques and recipes, and explore how incorporating cold press juices into your diet can enhance your overall well-being.

May this book be a guiding light on your journey towards salvation and wellness, reminding you of the profound link between the two and encouraging you to live a life that glorifies God in all aspects. May His grace and mercy accompany you every step of the way as you seek to honor Him with your whole being.

I have been juicing now for over two years and have found it to be a very beneficial way to help my body function, and provides a natural way to detox, as well as maintain a healthier diet. I balance juicing with regular meals, and this helps me to control my appetite as well as the desire to eat typically unhealthy food choices that only impart high cholesterols, and unhealthy additives.

Cold-pressed juicing can indeed be a great way to incorporate a variety of fruits and vegetables into your diet, providing essential nutrients and promoting overall health and wellbeing. The slow, gentle extraction method used in cold-pressed juicing helps retain more of the nutrients and enzymes present in the fruits and vegetables, making it a popular choice for those looking to maximize the health benefits of their juice. By incorporating cold-pressed juices into your routine along with a balanced diet and lifestyle, you can support your physical health while also embracing the principles of self-care and holistic well-being.

A healthy diet focused on fruits and vegetables, like juicing, can be aligned with the general principles of health and moderation found in various passages in the Bible. As the following devotional readings will convey there are great examples in the word of God. In Genesis 1:29, God gives fruits and plants for food to humans. Additionally, passages like 1
Corinthians 6:19-20 emphasize taking care of our bodies as they are temples of the Holy Spirit.
While juicing alone may not be explicitly mentioned in the Bible, the broader concept of nourishing our bodies with wholesome, plant based foods can be seen as aligning with biblical principles of health and stewardship.

"Be not wise in your own eyes; fear the Lord and turn away from evil. It will be healing to your flesh and refreshment to your bones." - Proverbs 3:7-8

This biblical statement emphasizes the importance of humility, respect for God, and staying away from harmful practices. By following a juicing diet that nourishes your body with essential nutrients and promotes good health, you can experience healing and refreshing effects that align with the principles of this passage.

DEVOTION 1: DANIEL'S EXAMPLE

In the book of Daniel, we find a powerful example of choosing a dietary path that honors God and promotes well-being. When faced with the temptation of indulging in the king's rich food and wine, Daniel and his companions made a bold decision to nourish their bodies with vegetables and water instead.

Their commitment to a plant-based diet, known today as the "Daniel Fast," demonstrates the importance of mindful eating and the impact it can have on our health. By choosing nutrient dense foods and abstaining from excessive indulgence, they honored God with their bodies and minds.

In the same way, as we embark on our juicing journey, may we be inspired by Daniel's devotion to God and his intentional choice of nourishing foods. Let us see juicing not just as a means of physical cleansing and renewal, but also as a form of spiritual discipline that aligns our bodies with God's design for health and vitality.

As we juice and partake in the goodness of fruits and vegetables, let us remember that our bodies are temples of the Holy Spirit,

(1 Corinthians 6:19-20). May every sip of juice be a reminder of our commitment to honoring God with our bodies and living a life that reflects gratitude for the gift of health and wellness. Amen.

DEVOTION 2: THE BODY IS OUR TEMPLE

In a world filled with tempting indulgences and unhealthy food choices, it can be challenging to prioritize our health and well-being. However, just as scripture guides us in matters of faith and morality, it also offers wisdom and guidance when it comes to caring for our bodies.

The Bible teaches us that our bodies are precious gifts from God, temples of the Holy Spirit (1 Corinthians 6:19-20). As stewards of these bodies, it is essential that we nurture and care for them with the same intentionality and reverence that we approach matters of the spirit.

One way we can honor God and steward our bodies well is through choosing to eat nourishing, wholesome foods that promote health and vitality. A healthy diet not only sustains our physical bodies but also impacts our mental clarity, emotional well-being, and spiritual connection.

Just as Jesus emphasized the importance of feeding the hungry and caring for those in need, we can show our love and gratitude for God's gift of health by making choices that prioritize nutritious and wholesome foods.

As you delve into the recipes within this book, may you be inspired to view healthy eating not as a chore or restriction, but as a joyful act of self-care and worship. May each meal you prepare be an opportunity to fuel your body, mind, and spirit with goodness and vitality.

Let us approach the table with thankfulness in our hearts, recognizing that every bite is a chance to honor God and cultivate a lifestyle of wholeness and well-being. May this recipe book serve as a guide and companion on your journey to nourishing your body and living a life that radiates God's love and grace. Amen.

DEVOTION 3: CREATED IN GOD'S IMAGE

As we embark on a mission of health and vitality through the art of juicing, let us take a moment to reflect on the profound significance of what we put into our bodies.

In the book of Genesis, we are reminded that God created us in His own image and entrusted us with the stewardship of our bodies (Genesis 1:27-28). Just as we are called to care for the earth and all living creatures, so too are we called to care for ourselves, honoring the sanctity of our bodies as vessels of His divine presence.

The act of juicing allows us to harness the abundance of fruits and vegetables that God has graciously provided for our nourishment. Through the process of extracting the vibrant liquid essence from these gifts of the earth, we can infuse our bodies with pure, concentrated nutrients that promote healing and vitality.

With each glass of freshly extracted juice, we are invited to partake in a sacred communion with nature and with God, honoring the wisdom of His creation and the miraculous power of natural foods to restore and rejuvenate our bodies.

Just as we cultivate and tend to a garden, so too must we cultivate and tend to our own inner gardens – the temple of our bodies – with love, care, and intention. Let us approach the juicing of fruits and vegetables not merely as a culinary endeavor, but as a spiritual practice that nourishes body, mind, and soul.

May the vibrant colors, flavors, and aromas of the juices we create remind us of the abundance of God's blessings and the infinite possibilities for health and healing that lie within His creation.

So, as you explore the juicing recipes in this booklet, may you be inspired to choose ingredients thoughtfully, with reverence for the wisdom and grace of God's design. May each sip of fresh juice be a reminder of the sacred connection between what we put in our bodies and the abundant life that He desires for us.
Amen.

DEVOTION 4: AN ATTITUDE OF GRATITUDE

Let us come together in gratitude for the gift of spiritual health, recognizing the importance of nourishing our souls and deepening our connection with the divine.

As we go through life, we encounter many challenges and distractions that can weigh heavily on our spirits. It is in these moments that we must turn inward, seeking solace and strength from the source of all comfort and peace.

Just as we prioritize physical health by nourishing our bodies with wholesome foods and exercise, let us also prioritize spiritual health by nourishing our souls with prayer, meditation, and acts of kindness.

In the book of Psalms, we are reminded of the restorative power of spending time in the presence of God. "He restores my soul; He leads me in the paths of righteousness for His name's sake." (Psalm 23:3) Let us take refuge in the arms of the Divine, allowing Him to renew and refresh our weary spirits.

Through prayer and meditation, we open our hearts to receive God's guidance and wisdom, finding solace in His presence and strength in His unfailing love. As we quiet our minds and listen for His voice, may we be reminded of the peace that surpasses all understanding, a peace that can only come from surrendering our worries and fears to Him.

Let us also seek spiritual health through acts of kindness and compassion towards others, embodying the love of God in all that we do. As we extend a helping hand to those in need, offer a listening ear to the lonely, and speak words of encouragement to the discouraged, we become channels of God's grace and instruments of His peace in the world.

In nurturing our spiritual health, may we be mindful of the interconnectedness of our body, mind, and spirit, understanding that true wellbeing encompasses all aspects of our being. Let us cultivate a daily practice of self-reflection, prayer, and service that honors the divine spark within us and encourages growth and transformation.

As we commit to prioritizing our spiritual health, may we be filled with a renewed sense of purpose and joy, knowing that we are walking in alignment with the divine will and experiencing the abundance of God's blessings. May our souls be nourished, our spirits uplifted, and our hearts open to receive the infinite love of our Creator. Amen.

DEVOTION 5: CELEBRATE LIFE

Let us rejoice in the abundance of life and the blessings of health that surround us each day. As we rejoice in the life God has provided, let our hearts overflow with joy for the gift of wellness and vitality that sustains us.

In the book of Psalms, we are reminded to "rejoice in the Lord always" (Philippians 4:4). Let us carry this message in our hearts as we celebrate the goodness of God's creation and the wonders of our own bodies, fearfully and wonderfully made.

With each breath we take, let us give thanks for the gift of life itself - for the beating of our hearts, the strength of our bodies, and the clarity of our minds. May we never take these blessings for granted, but instead cherish and nurture them with care and gratitude.

As we embark on this journey of health and wholeness, let us remember that true wellness encompasses not only the physical, but also the mental, emotional, and spiritual aspects of our being. Let us seek balance and harmony in all areas of our lives, striving to cultivate joy, peace, and contentment in each moment.

In nurturing our bodies, let us honor the sacred temple that houses our souls. May we fuel ourselves with nourishing foods, engage in physical activity that invigorates us, and rest and rejuvenate our spirits through adequate sleep and relaxation.

In caring for our minds, let us fill our thoughts with positivity and gratitude, casting out fear, doubt, and worry. Let us cultivate a spirit of optimism and resilience, knowing that a joyful heart is good medicine (Proverbs 17:22) that brings light and healing to our whole being.

In tending to our emotions, let us practice self-compassion and empathy towards ourselves and others. Let us embrace our feelings with love and acceptance, allowing ourselves to experience and express our emotions in healthy and constructive ways.

And in nourishing our spirits, let us cultivate a sense of connection with the divine source of all joy and peace. Let us seek solace and strength in prayer, meditation, and acts of kindness, knowing that as we draw near to God, He will draw near to us (James 4:8).

As we journey forward in pursuit of a healthy and vibrant life, may we be filled with a deep sense of gratitude and joy for every moment, every breath, and every opportunity to share our light with the world. May our lives be a testimony to the goodness and faithfulness of our Creator, who gifts us with the precious treasure of health and vitality.

With hearts overflowing with thanksgiving, let us lift up our voices in praise and declare: "This is the day that the Lord has made; let us rejoice and be glad in it" (Psalm 118:24). Amen.

DEVOTION 6: EMBRACING SALVATION AND WELLNESS

The transition into to salvation is a profound one, marked by the redemption and freedom offered to us through the sacrifice of Jesus Christ. In His love, we find forgiveness, reconciliation with God, and the promise of eternal life.

As we walk the path of salvation, let us also recognize the importance of caring for the temple of the Holy Spirit – our bodies. Just as we nurture our spiritual life through prayer and faith, let us also honor God by taking care of our physical well-being. Our bodies are fearfully and wonderfully made by the Creator, and we are called to steward them well.

In the pursuit of a healthy life, we are called to make choices that honor God by promoting wellness in body, mind, and spirit. This includes nourishing us with wholesome food, staying active, getting enough rest, and taking care of our mental and emotional health. By doing so, we reflect God's desire for us to live abundantly and serve Him with vitality and strength.

Let us remember that our bodies are instruments through which we can glorify God. By maintaining our health and well-being, we are better equipped to fulfill the purpose and calling that He has placed on our lives. Let us approach each day with gratitude for the gift of life and with a commitment to caring for ourselves in a way that honors Him.

As you read through the pages of this book, may you be inspired to embrace the connection between salvation and wellness. Let the message of God's love for you and His desire for your wholeness permeate your heart and soul. May you be empowered to make choices that align with His will and lead you towards a life of health, joy, and purpose. Amen.

DEVOTION 7: BEARING ONE ANOTHER'S BURDENS: A PATH TO SPIRITUAL AND SOCIAL HEALTH

The words of the apostle Paul in Galatians 6:2 remind us of the interconnectedness of our spiritual and social well-being. As followers of Christ, we are called to walk alongside one another, sharing in both the joys and struggles of life, and offering support and encouragement along the way.

In a world that often emphasizes individualism and self-sufficiency, the concept of bearing one another's burdens stands as a powerful testament to the transformative impact of community and relationship. When we willingly come alongside our brothers and sisters in Christ, offering a listening ear, a helping hand, or a heartfelt prayer, we create a space where spiritual and social health can flourish.

Just as a burden shared is a burden lightened, our willingness to empathize with and care for those around us not only strengthens our bonds of fellowship but also facilitates healing and growth in both the giver and receiver.

In lifting each other up, we reflect the love and compassion of Christ, embodying His teachings and fulfilling His command to love one another as He has loved us.

As we serve together in faith, let us be mindful of the opportunities we must bear one another's burdens. Whether it be through a simple act of kindness, a word of encouragement, or a heartfelt prayer, let us seek to support and uplift those around us, cultivating a culture of care and compassion that promotes spiritual and social flourishing.

In embracing the call to bear one another's burdens, we not only demonstrate our commitment to following Christ's example but also create a community where all are valued, heard, and cherished. May we be known for our love, our empathy, and our willingness to walk alongside one another in both the joys and challenges of life.

As we reflect on the words of Galatians 6:2, may we be inspired to actively participate in the journey of others, bearing their burdens with grace and humility, and in doing so, fulfilling the law of Christ. May our actions reflect His selfless love and our relationships be a testament to the transformative power of community and empathy. Amen.

DEVOTION 8: CULTIVATING A MINDSET OF EXCELLENCE

Finally, brothers and sisters, whatever is true, whatever is noble, whatever is right, whatever is pure, whatever is lovely, whatever is admirable— if anything is excellent or praiseworthy—think about such things." - Philippians 4:8 (NIV)

During our busy lives, it is easy to get caught up in negativity and discouragement. The world bombards us with messages that can weigh us down and distract us from the truth and goodness that surrounds us. However, as followers of Christ, we are called to a different way of thinking, one that is rooted in positivity, excellence, and gratitude.

The apostle Paul, in his letter to the Philippians, reminds us of the power of our thoughts and emotions. He encourages us to focus on things that are true, noble, right, pure, lovely, and praiseworthy. By intentionally directing our minds towards positivity and goodness, we can cultivate a mindset that reflects the character of Christ and brings light and hope into our lives and the lives of others.

Building positive habits of mind begins with intentionality and discipline. It requires us to be mindful of the content we allow into our minds, whether through media, conversations, or our own internal dialogue. By choosing to dwell on thoughts that uplift and inspire, we not only strengthen our own spiritual life but also radiate joy and encouragement to those around us.

As we meditate on the words of Philippians 4:8, let us be challenged to examine our thought patterns and habits. Are we nurturing a mindset of excellence, focusing on the goodness and beauty that God has placed before us? Or are we allowing negative thoughts and beliefs to cloud our perception and hinder our growth?

Let us strive to cultivate habits of mind that reflect the characteristics outlined in Philippians 4:8. May we seek out truth in a world of deception, honor in a culture of disregard, purity in a society of moral decline, and beauty in a world of brokenness. As we fix our thoughts on the things that are excellent and praiseworthy, may we discover the transformative power of positive thinking in our lives and the lives of those around us.

In embracing a mindset of excellence, we not only draw closer to the heart of God but also inspire others to do the same. May our thoughts be a reflection of His grace and love, pointing others towards the source of all goodness and truth. May our habits of mind lead us to a deeper relationship with Christ and a life filled with purpose, hope, and joy. Amen.

May this devotion inspire you to reflect on the power of positive thinking and encourage you to cultivate habits that elevate your mindset towards excellence and goodness. Amen.

DEVOTION 9: BUILDING A HEALTHY COMMUNITY AND FAMILY

Romans 12:5 (NIV) - "so in Christ we, though many, form one body, and each member belongs to all the others."

As followers of Christ, we are called to be a part of a community where we support and care for one another as a family. Just as the Scripture says, "we, though many, form one body" in Christ, highlighting the interconnectedness and importance of unity in our relationships.

Appreciating Diversity: God has created each one of us uniquely with different gifts, talents, and perspectives. In a healthy community and family, we celebrate this diversity and recognize the value that each individual brings to the whole. How can we embrace and appreciate the differences within our community, understanding that we are all essential parts of God's plan?

Mutual Care and Support: In a thriving community, we look out for one another, offering help, encouragement, and prayers in times of need. Reflect on ways you can actively support and uplift your community members, just as you would for your own family. How can we extend the love of

Christ through our actions and words towards those in our community?

Shared Purpose and Mission: As members of the body of Christ, we are united in our purpose of spreading His love and message to the world. Think about how your community and family can work together to fulfill this mission. How can we serve others, share the gospel, and be a light in our community, demonstrating God's love through our unity and actions?

Prayer: Let us pray for our community and family, asking God to strengthen the bonds of love and unity among us. May we be guided by His Spirit to build healthy relationships, support one another in times of joy and trial, and glorify Him through our shared mission.

As we reflect on the importance of building a healthy community and family rooted in Christ, let us strive to practice love, unity, and mutual care in all our relationships. Together, let us be a shining example of God's love in this world.
Amen.

DEVOTION 10: GUIDED BY FAITH

Scripture Reference: Proverbs 3:5-6 (NIV) - "Trust in the Lord with all your heart and lean not on your own understanding; in all your ways submit to him, and he will make your paths straight."

Life is filled with twists and turns, highs and lows, challenges, and triumphs. Along this journey, we may face uncertainties and doubts about the path ahead. However, we are reminded in Proverbs 3:5-6 to trust in the Lord with all our hearts and lean not on our own understanding. This verse reminds us that our faith should be a guiding light in our journey of life.

Trusting in the Lord involves surrendering our worries, fears, and doubts to Him. It requires us to have faith that God will guide us through any challenges we may face. When we put our trust in Him, we can experience peace and assurance that He will lead us in the right direction.

As we navigate the ups and downs of life, it is important to seek God's guidance in all our decisions. By submitting to Him in all our ways, we can rest assured that He will make our paths straight. God's wisdom surpasses our own understanding, and when we follow His direction, we can be alert, focused, and revitalized throughout the day.

Weight Management: Cold press juices can be a convenient way to incorporate more fruits and vegetables into your diet, promoting satiety and helping you maintain a healthy weight over time.

confident that He will lead us to where we need to be.

Let us trust in the Lord wholeheartedly as we make our way through life. May we lean on His wisdom and guidance, knowing that He is with us every step of the way. As we surrender our lives to Him, may we experience the peace and comfort that comes from following His path for us. Amen.

1.

UNDERSTANDING COLD PRESS JUICING

Cold press juicing has gained popularity in recent years for its ability to preserve nutrients and produce fresh, flavorful juices. In this chapter, we will delve into what cold press juicing is, how it differs from other juicing methods, and the various benefits it offers for your health and wellness.

What is Cold Press Juicing?
Cold press juicing, also known as slow juicing or masticating juicing, is a method of extracting juice from fruits and vegetables using a gentle, slow process. Unlike traditional centrifugal juicers that rely on high-speed spinning blades to extract juice, cold press juicers utilize a hydraulic press or auger to slowly crush and squeeze the produce, minimizing heat and oxidation in the process.

How Does Cold Press Juicing Differ from Other Juicing Methods?
One of the key differences between cold press juicing and other juicing methods, such as centrifugal juicing, is the manner in which the juice is extracted. Cold press juicers operate at lower speeds and with less heat, resulting in minimal exposure to air and oxidation. This helps to preserve the

enzymes, vitamins, and minerals i‌
to a higher-quality drink that retain‌

Benefits of Cold Press Juicing for Hea‌
Wellness
There are several benefits to incorpor‌
juices into your diet, including:

1. Higher Nutrient Retention: The ge‌
   extraction process of cold press juic‌
   preserve the natural enzymes, vitam‌
   minerals found in fruits and vegetabl‌
   ensuring that you receive maximum n‌
   with every glass.

2. Improved Immune Function: Cold press ‌
   are rich in antioxidants and phytonutrien‌
   which can help to boost your immune sys‌
   fight inflammation, and protect against ch‌
   diseases.

3. Enhanced Digestion: The vitamins and miner‌
   in cold press juices can support digestive
   health by promoting regularity, aiding in
   nutrient absorption, and soothing gut
   inflammation.

4. Increased Energy Levels: Drinking cold press
   juices packed with nutrients can provide a
   natural energy boost, helping you feel more

2.

GETTING STARTED WITH COLD PRESS JUICING

Now that you have learned the basics of cold press juicing and the numerous health benefits it offers, it's time to dive into the practical aspect of getting started with this refreshing and nutritious practice. In this chapter, we will cover essential equipment and ingredients, tips for selecting and prepping produce, and guidelines for storing and consuming your cold press juices.

Essential Equipment for Cold Press Juicing
To embark on your cold press juicing journey, you will need the following essential equipment:

1. Cold Press Juicer: Invest in a high-quality cold press juicer to ensure optimal nutrient retention and juice quality. There are various models available, ranging from horizontal auger juicers to vertical masticating juicers. Choose a juicer that suits your budget, space, and juicing needs.

2. Cutting Board and Knife: A sharp knife and cutting board will be essential for slicing and chopping fruits and vegetables before juicing.

confident that He will lead us to where we need to be.

Let us trust in the Lord wholeheartedly as we make our way through life. May we lean on His wisdom and guidance, knowing that He is with us every step of the way. As we surrender our lives to Him, may we experience the peace and comfort that comes from following His path for us. Amen.

1.
UNDERSTANDING COLD PRESS JUICING

Cold press juicing has gained popularity in recent years for its ability to preserve nutrients and produce fresh, flavorful juices. In this chapter, we will delve into what cold press juicing is, how it differs from other juicing methods, and the various benefits it offers for your health and wellness.

What is Cold Press Juicing?
Cold press juicing, also known as slow juicing or masticating juicing, is a method of extracting juice from fruits and vegetables using a gentle, slow process. Unlike traditional centrifugal juicers that rely on high-speed spinning blades to extract juice, cold press juicers utilize a hydraulic press or auger to slowly crush and squeeze the produce, minimizing heat and oxidation in the process.

How Does Cold Press Juicing Differ from Other Juicing Methods?
One of the key differences between cold press juicing and other juicing methods, such as centrifugal juicing, is the manner in which the juice is extracted. Cold press juicers operate at lower speeds and with less heat, resulting in minimal exposure to air and oxidation. This helps to preserve the

enzymes, vitamins, and minerals in the juice, leading to a higher-quality drink that retains more nutrients.

Benefits of Cold Press Juicing for Health and Wellness

There are several benefits to incorporating cold press juices into your diet, including:

1. Higher Nutrient Retention: The gentle extraction process of cold press juicing helps to preserve the natural enzymes, vitamins, and minerals found in fruits and vegetables, ensuring that you receive maximum nutrition with every glass.

2. Improved Immune Function: Cold press juices are rich in antioxidants and phytonutrients, which can help to boost your immune system, fight inflammation, and protect against chronic diseases.

3. Enhanced Digestion: The vitamins and minerals in cold press juices can support digestive health by promoting regularity, aiding in nutrient absorption, and soothing gut inflammation.

4. Increased Energy Levels: Drinking cold press juices packed with nutrients can provide a natural energy boost, helping you feel more

alert, focused, and revitalized throughout the day.

5. Weight Management: Cold press juices can be a convenient way to incorporate more fruits and vegetables into your diet, promoting satiety and helping you maintain a healthy weight over time.

3.

JUICING TECHNIQUES AND RECIPES FOR COLD PRESS JUICING

In this chapter, we will explore the art of cold press juicing, a method that preserves the nutrients and enzymes in fruits and vegetables better than traditional juicing techniques. Cold press juicing involves slowly extracting juice from produce using hydraulic pressure, resulting in a higher-quality juice that retains more of the vitamins, minerals, and antioxidants present in the ingredients. Let's dive into the step-by-step process of cold press juicing, tips for mixing and matching ingredients for delicious flavor combinations, and how to adjust juice consistency and sweetness to suit your preferences.

Step-by-Step Guide to Cold Press Juicing:

1. Prepare Your Ingredients: Wash and chop your fruits and vegetables into small pieces that are easy to feed into the juicer chute.

2. Assemble Your Cold Press Juicer: Set up your cold press juicer according to the manufacturer's instructions, ensuring that all components are securely in place.

3.   Begin Juicing: Start by feeding a small handful of produce into the juicer at a time, allowing the machine to slowly extract the juice.

4.   Mix and Match Ingredients: Get creative with your cold press juice recipes by combining different fruits, vegetables, and herbs. Consider flavor combinations that complement each other and provide a variety of nutrients.

5.   Adjust Consistency and Sweetness: To customize your juice to your liking, you can adjust the consistency by adding more water or reducing the amount of pulp. You can also sweeten your juice with fruits like apples or pears if desired.

6.   Serve and Enjoy: Once you've finished juicing, pour the fresh juice into a glass and savor its vibrant colors and flavors. Drink immediately to maximize the benefits of the live enzymes present in the juice.

7.   Clean Your Cold Press Juicer: After juicing, disassemble the juicer and clean each component thoroughly to ensure optimal performance and hygiene for future juicing sessions.

Mixing and Matching Ingredients for Delicious Flavor Combinations:

- Citrus Delight: Mix oranges, grapefruits, and a splash of lemon for a bright and zesty juice packed with Vitamin C.
- Green Goddess: Combine kale, spinach, cucumber, and green apples for a refreshing and nutrient-dense green juice.
- Tropical Paradise: Blend pineapple, mango, coconut water, and a hint of mint for a tropical themed juice that transports you to an island getaway.

Adjusting Juice Consistency and Sweetness to Suit Your Preferences:

- For a thicker juice, reduce the amount of water added during the juicing process.
- To sweeten your juice, add naturally sweet fruits like berries, bananas, or pineapple.
- Adjust the flavor profile by incorporating herbs like mint, basil, or cilantro for a fresh and invigorating twist.

By mastering cold press juicing techniques, experimenting with different ingredients, and customizing your juice to suit your preferences, you can enjoy a wide range of delicious and nutritious beverages that support your health and well-being. Stay tuned for more tips and insights on how to elevate your cold press juicing experience and make the most of this beneficial practice in your daily routine. Cheers to vibrant health and vibrant flavors!

4.

HEALTH BENEFITS OF COLD PRESS JUICING: CLEANSING AND DETOXING

Some of the Health Benefits of Cold Press Juicing is that it helps keep acid out of the body, provides a healthier digestion system, can adjust body systems that reduce the need for certain medications.

Juice cleansing and detoxing have become popular practices for improving health, promoting weight loss, and resetting the body. In this chapter, we will explore the benefits of juice cleansing and detoxing with cold press juicing, as well as provide guidance on how to incorporate these practices into your healthy lifestyle.

Benefits of Juice Cleansing and Detoxing

Juice cleansing and detoxing involve consuming only fresh juices made from fruits, vegetables, and herbs for a period of time, typically ranging from one to several days. This practice allows the body to rest and recharge while flooding it with vital nutrients and antioxidants. Some of the potential benefits of juice cleansing and detoxing include:

1. Improved Digestion: Juices are easier for the body to digest and absorb, giving the digestive

system a break and potentially reducing bloating and gas.

2. Increased Energy: By eliminating processed foods and focusing on nutrient-dense juices, you may experience a boost in energy levels and mental clarity.

3. Weight Loss: Juice cleansing can kickstart weight loss by reducing calorie intake and cleansing the body of toxins that may contribute to weight gain.

4. Detoxification: Cold press juices are rich in antioxidants and phytonutrients that support the body's natural detoxification processes, helping to eliminate toxins and waste from the body. 5. Enhanced Nutrient Intake: Juicing allows you to consume a variety of fruits and vegetables in concentrated form, providing vital vitamins, minerals, and antioxidants that support overall health.

Incorporating Juice Cleansing and Detoxing

If you're interested in trying a juice cleanse or detox, here are some tips for incorporating it into your routine:

1. Start Slow: If you're new to juice cleansing, consider starting with a one-day cleanse and gradually increasing the duration as you become more comfortable with the process. 2. Choose High-Quality Ingredients: Use organic fruits and vegetables whenever possible to minimize exposure to pesticides and chemicals.

3. Stay Hydrated: In addition to consuming juices, drink plenty of water throughout the day to stay hydrated and help flush out toxins.

4. Listen to Your Body: Pay attention to how you feel during the cleanse and adjust as needed. If you experience dizziness, weakness, or other adverse effects, stop the cleanse and consult a healthcare professional.

5. Transition Back to Solid Foods: After completing a cleanse, slowly reintroduce solid foods into your diet to avoid digestive discomfort. Start with lighter, easily digestible foods and fruits like, watermelon, salads and soups.

By incorporating juice cleansing and detoxing with cold press juicing into your routine, you can support your overall health and well-being while discovering the transformative power of fresh, nutrient-dense juices. In the next chapter, I will provide tips on incorporating juicing into a long term healthy lifestyle for sustained benefits. Stay tuned for more insights on your cold press juicing journey.

5.
RECIPES FOR COLD PRESS JUICES

In this chapter, we will explore a selection of delicious and nutritious recipes for cold press juices. These blends of fruits, vegetables, herbs, and superfoods are designed to provide a boost of essential vitamins, minerals, and antioxidants while tantalizing your taste buds. Let's dive into these refreshing and health-enhancing creations that you can easily prepare with your cold press juicer.

1. Green Detox Elixir
-     Ingredients: 2 large handfuls of kale, 1 cucumber, 2 celery stalks, 1 green apple, 1 lemon
(peeled), 1 inch piece of ginger
-     Instructions: Feed all the ingredients through the cold press juicer, starting with the leafy greens. Stir well and pour into a glass. This vibrant green juice is packed with detoxifying nutrients to help cleanse your body and boost your energy levels.

2. Berry Blast Antioxidant Juice -
Ingredients:
1 cup of mixed berries (such as strawberries, blueberries, raspberries), 1 beet, 1 orange

(peeled), Handful of mint leaves

- Instructions: Juice the berries, beet, and orange together. Add in the mint leaves at the end for a refreshing finish. This antioxidant-rich juice is bursting with flavor and immune-boosting properties.

3. Immune-Boosting Citrus Sunshine Juice

- Ingredients: 2 oranges (peeled), 2 carrots 1 lemon (peeled), 1 inch piece of turmeric root

- Instructions: Juice the oranges, carrots, and lemon, then add the turmeric root for an extra anti-inflammatory kick. This bright and zesty juice is perfect for supporting your immune system and uplifting your mood.

4. Pineapple Paradise Tropical Juice -

Ingredients:

1 cup of pineapple chunks

1 mango

1 kiwi

Handful of spinach

Coconut water (to taste)

- Instructions: Combine the pineapple, mango, kiwi, and spinach, then blend with coconut water to your preferred consistency. This tropical infused juice is packed with vitamins, minerals, and hydration for a refreshing sip of paradise.

5. Cool Cucumber Mint Cleanser
-    Ingredients: 1 cucumber, Handful of mint leaves, 1 green apple, 1 lemon (peeled)
-    Instructions: Juice the cucumber, mint leaves, green apple, and lemon together. This soothing and hydrating juice is perfect for a refreshing cleanse and to promote healthy digestion.

6. Citrus Ginger Blast
- Ingredients: Oranges, Ginger
- Instructions: Juice the oranges and ginger together for a zesty and tangy juice that will give you a Vitamin C boost.

7. Tropical Paradise
- Ingredients: Pineapple, Apples, Pears
- Instructions: Juice the pineapple, apples, and pears for a tropical and sweet juice that is perfect for summer.

8. Sweet Melon Medley
- Ingredients: Watermelon, Cantaloupe, Honeydew Melon
- Instructions: Juice the watermelon, cantaloupe, and honeydew melon together for a hydrating and refreshing drink.

9. Cherry Berry Burst
- Ingredients: Cherries, Mixed Berries

- Instructions: Juice the cherries and mixed berries for a flavorful and antioxidant-rich juice that is bursting with goodness.

10. Green Power
   - Ingredients: Celery, Kale, Granny Apples
   - Instructions: Juice the celery, kale, and Granny apples for a green juice that is packed with nutrients and will give you an energy boost.

11. Carrot Zinger
   - Ingredients: Carrots, Oranges, Ginger
   - Instructions: Juice the carrots, oranges, and ginger for a zingy and vitamin-packed juice that is great for boosting your immune system.

12. Turmeric Tonic
   - Ingredients: Carrots, Turmeric, Oranges, Lemon
   - Instructions: Juice the carrots, turmeric, oranges, and lemon for a anti-inflammatory and immune-boosting tonic that will also give you a dose of Vitamin C.

13. Berry Blast
   - Ingredients: Blueberries, Raspberries, Blackberries, Strawberries

- Instructions: Juice the mixed berries for a delicious and antioxidant-rich juice that is bursting with flavor.

14. Pineapple Mint Refresher
   - Ingredients: Pineapple, Mint Leaves, Lime
   - Instructions: Juice the pineapple, mint leaves, and lime for a refreshing and zesty drink that is perfect for a hot day.

15. Cucumber Cooler
   - Ingredients: Cucumber, Celery, Green Apples, Mint Leaves
   - Instructions: Juice the cucumber, celery, green apples, and mint leaves for a cooling and hydrating juice that is perfect for detoxifying.

16. Citrus Cleanser
   - Ingredients: Oranges, Grapefruits, Lemons, Ginger
   - Instructions: Juice the oranges, grapefruits, lemons, and some ginger for a refreshing and cleansing juice that is full of Vitamin C.

17. Beet Blast
   - Ingredients: Beets, Carrots, Apples, Lemons
   - Instructions: Juice the beets, carrots, apples, and lemons for a vibrant and nutrient-rich juice that is great for detoxification.

18. Tropical Paradise
-    Ingredients: Pineapple, Mango, Kiwi, Coconut Water
-    Instructions: Juice the pineapple, mango, and kiwi, then mix with coconut water for a tropical and hydrating juice that feels like a vacation in a glass.

19. Green Goddess
- Ingredients: Spinach, Cucumber, Green Apples, Celery, Lemon
- Instructions: Juice the spinach, cucumber, green apples, celery, and lemon for a green powerhouse juice that is loaded with vitamins and minerals.

20. Watermelon Wonder
- Ingredients: Watermelon, Strawberries, Mint Leaves, Lime
- Instructions: Juice the watermelon and strawberries, then blend with mint leaves and lime for a refreshing and hydrating juice that is perfect for hot summer days.

21. Spicy Sunrise
- Ingredients: Carrots, Oranges, Turmeric, Cayenne Pepper
- Instructions: Juice carrots and oranges, then add a dash of turmeric and cayenne pepper for a

spicy and invigorating juice that is great for boosting immunity.

22. Beyond Berry Blast

- Ingredients: Blueberries, Raspberries, Blackberries, Almond Milk, Honey
- Instructions: Blend blueberries, raspberries, blackberries, and almond milk with a touch of honey for a delicious and antioxidant-rich berry smoothie.

23. Golden Glow

- Ingredients: Pineapple, Yellow Bell Pepper, Ginger, Lemon
- Instructions: Juice pineapple, yellow bell pepper, ginger, and lemon for a sunny and vibrant juice that is filled with Vitamin C and anti-inflammatory properties.

24. Beach Breeze

- Ingredients: Watermelon, Cucumber, Mint, Coconut Water
- Instructions: Blend watermelon, cucumber, mint, and coconut water for a refreshing and hydrating juice that feels like a cool breeze on a hot day.

25. Choco-Banana Bliss

- Ingredients: Bananas, Almond Milk, Cacao Powder, Dates

- Instructions: Blend bananas, almond milk, cacao powder, and dates for a decadent and chocolaty smoothie that is rich in potassium and antioxidants.

These recipes offer a mix of flavors and textures to keep your juicing experience exciting and satisfying. Enjoy trying out these diverse juice creations!

Feel free to experiment with these recipes, adjust ingredient quantities to suit your taste preferences, and explore your creativity in crafting your own cold press juice blends. Cheers to vibrant health and flavorful sips of goodness!

6.

INCORPORATING JUICING INTO A LONG-TERM HEALTHY LIFESTYLE

In Chapter 4, we explored the benefits of juice cleansing and detoxing with cold press juicing. In this chapter, we will focus on how to incorporate juicing into a long-term healthy lifestyle for sustained benefits and overall well-being.

Juicing can be a powerful tool for increasing your intake of essential nutrients, promoting hydration, and supporting overall health. By incorporating fresh juices into your daily routine, you can nourish your body, boost your energy levels, and enhance your overall vitality. Here are some tips for incorporating juicing into a long-term healthy lifestyle:

1. Make it a Daily Habit: Aim to include a fresh juice in your daily routine, whether as a morning pick-me-up, an afternoon snack, or as part of your meals. By making juicing a consistent habit, you can reap the benefits of ongoing nutrient intake.

2. Experiment with Different Combinations: Get creative with your juicing recipes by trying out different combinations of fruits, vegetables, and herbs. Mixing and matching ingredients can help

keep things exciting and ensure you get a varied range of nutrients.

3. Plan Ahead: To make juicing convenient, consider prepping ingredients in advance. Wash, chop, and portion out fruits and vegetables so that when it's time to juice, you can quickly assemble your ingredients and enjoy a fresh and nutritious drink.

4. Drink Mindfully: Take the time to savor and enjoy your fresh juice. Practice mindfulness by being present in the moment while you drink, acknowledging the nourishment and energy it provides to your body.

5. Supplement with Solid Foods: While juicing can be a valuable addition to your diet, it's essential to complement it with whole foods to ensure you're getting a balanced intake of nutrients, including fiber and protein.

6. Listen to Your Body: Pay attention to how your body responds to juicing and adjust your intake as needed. If you feel bloated or experience digestive discomfort, consider incorporating more vegetables and reducing the fruit content in your juices.

7. Stay Consistent: Consistency is key to reaping the long-term benefits of juicing. Make juicing a lasting part of your healthy lifestyle by integrating it into your daily routine and prioritizing your well-being.

By incorporating juicing into a long-term healthy lifestyle, you can enhance your nutritional intake, support your health goals, and enjoy the benefits of fresh, nutrient-dense juices on a regular basis. Stay tuned for more tips and insights on how to make juicing a sustainable and enjoyable practice in your everyday life.
Cheers to your health and vitality!

7.

TYPES OF JUICERS

There are several types of juicers available on the market, each with their own pros and cons. Here are some popular types of juicers and their characteristics:

1. Centrifugal Juicers: These juicers are typically more affordable and work by using a fast-spinning blade to extract juice from fruits and vegetables. They are quick and efficient but may produce less juice from leafy greens and harder produce.

2. Masticating Juicers (Slow Juicers): These juicers operate at a slower speed, which helps retain more nutrients in the juice. They can effectively juice leafy greens, hard produce, and even nuts. Although they are slower than centrifugal juicers, many people appreciate the nutrient-rich juice they produce.

3. Citrus Juicers: Designed specifically for juicing citrus fruits like oranges, lemons, and limes, these juicers are easy to use and extract juice efficiently.

4. Triturating Juicers (Twin-Gear Juicers): These juicers use two gears to crush produce and extract juice. They are known for producing high-quality juice with maximum nutrition, but they can be more expensive and time-consuming to clean.

When choosing a juicer, consider factors such as the types of produce you will be juicing, ease of cleaning, juice quality, and your budget. Ultimately, the best kind of juicer for you will depend on your personal juicing preferences and needs.

8.
THE ADVANTAGE OF THE COLD PRESS JUICER

Cold press juicers, which is the type that I prefer are also known as masticating or slow juicers, have several benefits compared to other types of juicers like centrifugal juicers. Here are some advantages of cold press juicers:

1. Better Juice Quality: Cold press juicers operate at a slower speed, which reduces heat and oxidation during the juicing process. This helps retain more nutrients, enzymes, and antioxidants in the juice, resulting in a higher quality juice that is fresher and more vibrant.

2. Higher Juice Yield: Cold press juicers typically extract more juice from the same amount of produce compared to centrifugal juicers. The slow, efficient extraction process ensures that you get the most out of your fruits and vegetables, producing a higher juice yield and reducing food waste.

3. Juice Storage: Cold press juicers produce juice that lasts longer due to the reduced oxidation.

This means you can store your juice for up to 72 hours without significant loss of nutrients and flavor. This is especially beneficial if you like to make juice in bulk or prefer to prepare juice in advance.

4. Versatility: Cold press juicers are versatile and can effectively juice a wide variety of produce, including leafy greens, hard vegetables, and even nuts for nut milk. Their slow and powerful extraction process can handle a range of ingredients, making them ideal for creating nutrient-rich and flavorful juices.

5. Cold Press Juicers provide a very efficient juicing experience while at the same time being higher in quality and available at most health food outlets, and department or appliance stores.

While cold press juicers may have a higher price point and slower juicing process compared to centrifugal juicers, many people believe that the superior juice quality and nutritional benefits justify the investment. Ultimately, the choice of juicer will depend on your personal preferences and juicing needs.

CONCLUSION

Since I have been dedicated to juicing, I have experienced its numerous benefits firsthand. Not only has juicing proven to be an effective way to support my body's functions and aid in natural detoxification, but it has also helped me maintain a healthier diet overall.

By incorporating juicing into my routine alongside regular meals, I have been able to better control my appetite and reduce cravings for unhealthy, high-cholesterol food choices. Juicing has truly become a cornerstone of my wellness journey, transforming the way I nourish and care for my body.

As you reach the end of "Cold Press Juicing: A Comprehensive Guide to Health and Wellness," I hope you feel inspired and empowered to embrace the spiritual and physical benefits of this devotional and guide.

I hope this guide helps you create delicious and nutritious cold press juices to support your health and well-being. Happy juicing, and Cheers to a healthier you!

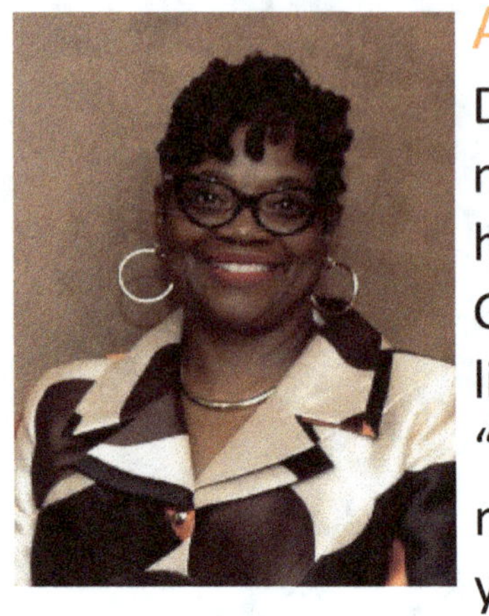

ABOUT THE AUTHOR

Daphne Gresham-Gaddy is a mother and grandmother who has raised her children to value God and live healthy abundant lives. She is a pastor's daughter, "PK" and has served as a ministry wife for over twenty years. Coming from a career of being a licensed cosmetologist instructor, she now leads women's ministry and seeks to impart others with healthy spiritual empowerment as well as a healthy way to live. Having served as a Certified Church Planting Wives Encourager, she speaks and serves women in ministry all over the nation.

May this juicing devotional and recipe book serve as a tool for us to honor God through the care and stewardship of our bodies. Let us juice with intention, gratitude, and mindfulness, knowing that every glass of fresh juice is an opportunity to nourish our bodies, honor God, and embrace a lifestyle of wholeness and wellbeing. Amen.

- "Lady G"